Redeem Your Health

A 21-Day Cleanse and Detox Jumpstart

by Dr. Angie Welikala

Printed in the United States of America

Made to Heal, Dr. Angie Welikala

www.madetoheal.com

Disclaimer: This book was written as a guide to assist my patients as they conduct the detox and cleanse while in my care. This book is only to be used by persons conducting the detox and cleanse under the supervision of a licensed healthcare professional. The supplements and products in this book are products I use and recommend to my patients. I am in no way affiliated with nor paid by the companies who produce or distribute the products.

While we carry Standard Process products, neither Dr. Angie Welikala nor any third party associated with, related to, or linked to Dr. Angie Welikala's business or website is in any way affiliated with Standard Process Inc.® Standard Process expressly disclaims any responsibility for, and makes no representations or warranties regarding, any statement, information, materials, or content found on or included in Dr. Angie Welikala's marketing materials/website, or any third party marketing materials/websites related to, associated with or linked to Dr. Angie Welikala's business or website. Standard Process products are dietary supplements and not intended to diagnose, treat, cure, or prevent any disease.

Bible Translation Copyright Information

ISBN-13: 978-0-615-74382-0

ISBN-10: 061574382X

First Edition, January 2013

10 9 8 7 6 5 4 3 2

Redeem Your Health

Dear Molly,

Thank you for being my sponsor and my new Sister in Christ! Love you to the Moon & Back!

Dr. Angela

8-23-15

What People Are Saying

"Dr Angie Welikala has written a beautiful how-to guide on reclaiming your health and your life! I love this book! Her simple methods result in not just a strong, healthy body but a renewed spirit."

- Cynthia Pasquella, CCN, Celebrity Nutritionist and Best-Selling Author of The Hungry Hottie Cookbook

"If there is one thing I learned, this cleanse has taught me to incorporate more greens and veggies into every meal. I am not perfect, and if I have a bite of something, it's not the end of the world. This has kept me focused."

—Shelby W.

"The Lord has truly blessed me in helping me find Dr. Angie. Dr. Angie not only helps you heal physically, but mentally and emotionally as well. She is such an amazing person! Dr. Angie you are the bomb!"

—Babette P.

"Great motivation. Felt like you were right there with me."

—Shelly C.

"The daily inspiration from you made it easier to keep on track and not to feel like a failure if you get a little off track. JUST MOVE ON. Very KEY for me to remember! I made LIFE changes not just a few days of change!"

—Amy B.

"Dr. Angie Welikala is a Wonder Woman, strongly Christian based, and I wouldn't be moving my head or have less back pain if I wasn't a patient of hers. I was involved in a propane tank explosion which caused trauma to my body. When I first started seeing her as my doctor I was totally unable to move my neck or head AT ALL. Within two weeks I was able to move and drive. Now, I cannot imagine my life without her as my chiropractor! Thank you Dr. Angie Welikala for helping my body heal! You're amazing! Always your patient,"

—Cathie C.

"Dr. Welikala has created a great and compelling detoxification program that is both effective and thought-provoking. Her prayerful process made it spiritually healing as well. I enjoyed it and highly recommend it."

—-Dr. Danita Thomas Heagy

"There are many voices today talking about detoxing. Dr. Angie Welikala is one of only a very few emphasizing the importance of doing a gentle physical, emotional, and spiritual detox all at the same time. (In a way that fits with both my busy schedule and my budget!) Thank you Dr. Angie!"

—Jeannie Burlowski, Owner, www.getintomedicalschool.com.

"I started reading Dr. Angie's 21-Day cleanse blog, not because I was doing the cleanse, but because I am on the mailing list. But here's what happened! As she motivated daily about strength, courage, commitment and perseverance—tying her words into scripture—I too started to change some of my 'not so healthy' eating behaviors! Dr. Angie's blog seemed to be in tune with how the group may have felt at any given moment as she blogged about temptations and drawbacks, all the while keeping the focus, letting God's words and strength be your guide. As the group finished up, the blog continued sharing about the weaknesses of self, self-destructive behaviors, guilt, as well as the let down of a once strong community disbanding. Dr. Angie kept us strong through the help of God on this journey, not once letting us down, or dishonoring us with our human weakness. Although this blog is supposed to be about a simple 21-Day cleanse, I think it is WAY more far-reaching than that. It is a must read for anybody with a personal goal. Thank you Dr. Angie!"

—Dr. Muffit Jensen, Burbank, CA

"You really teach us how to make better health choices. All the extra classes and information you offer have been very informative. I feel great!"

—Cathy M.

"I had a slight headache, but that went away after a couple days. I felt really good throughout the detox and lost approximately 8 lbs. Try it and just take it day by day. You are stronger than you think you are and you will feel much better than you thought you would."

—Nancy, M.

"Dr. Angie, I want to THANK YOU for the opportunity to be part of the detox program. Your daily email filled with encouragement, transparency, and brutal honesty were REFRESHING and had a way of zeroing in on everything I was experiencing! It was important to me to know that I was part of a group striving for the same goal, experiencing the same struggle or victory . . . I knew I wasn't alone! With MUCH love & appreciation."

—Lanette Sperline

~ As iron sharpens iron, so people can improve each other. ~

Proverbs 27:17 [ncv]

"I was grateful to have daily encouragement, education, and support while learning a new and healthier way of eating."

—Kris S.

"For anyone truly interested in redeeming their health from the chronic diseases that so many are burdened with today, Dr. Welikala has written an easy-to-read 'how to' practical guide that could provide life and wellness for you and your family."

—Diana Noland, MPH RD CCN, Integrative and Functional Medical Nutrition Therapy, Adjunct Faculty, U of Kansas Medical Center, www.nolandnutrition.com

"Dr. Angie Welikala has created a well-thought-out, comprehensive detox program that will reset your body and promote emotional and physical well-being. Dr. Angie Welikala has taken the body and mind as a whole for the most effective detoxification one can achieve. She is your biggest cheerleader and supporter throughout this whole program, which really encourages you to succeed! Thank you for letting me be a part of this wonderful program."

—Tawny Lovett
www.shophealingheart.com

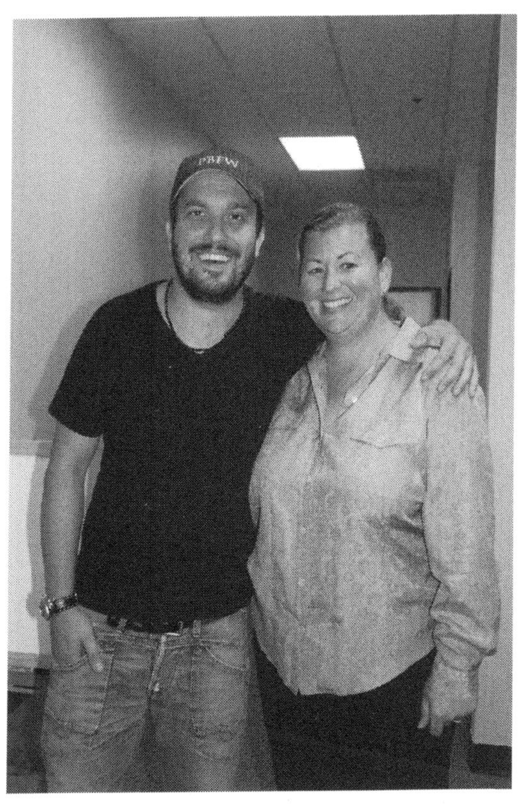

By the end 2012, I had traveled out of Los Angeles for 287 days amounting to over 170 flights and about 320,000 fly miles, (yes, I have Diamond Status with ALL the Airlines) and I have done approximately 130,000 Miles with in my car. Can you imagine how my back felt? Did I mention that I also get up at 5 a.m. and never go to bed till about 1 a.m. everyday, 7 days a week? I often forget to eat during the day and I find myself chewing Italian cold cuts and cheeses in my bed right before I sleep. My life was a mess and my back was killing me. Then, I met Doctor Angie. She gave me a hug and she told me, 'Dude, just relax, take sometime for yourself. What's wrong with you?' She did her magic on my back and now my two bulging discs (one going left, one going right, yes seriously) are actually not bothering me much anymore. I feel blessed to be in Dr. Angie's care. She is truly committed to her patient's well-being and listens when concerns are shared and offers guidance and explanations beyond the profession she performs. She knows that healing takes place on all levels—physical, emotional, mental, and spiritual. That is why her cleanse program is so great. It shows you to cleanse more than food; you cleanse every part of yourself for full healing.

Doctor Angie is like a friend I feel comfortable to listen to because I know she has my best interests at heart. Besides my mom, she is the only person I ever meet that told me, "I'll pray for you while you are traveling" . . . and that's good business. Did I mention already that she is a hell of a Chiropractor? And I mean it in the best way possible. She should charge me five times what she does but I'm thankful she doesn't. :-)

Angie you're the best, and thank you for squeezing me in your studio always at the worse time of the day to accommodate my schedule.

I appreciate it, much Love!
Chef Fabio Viviani

Check out what's going on at www.fabioviviani.com!

Acknowledgements

First and foremost, I give Glory to God for all He has done in the creation of this book. Thank you, family and friends who have been part of this journey and part of this detox and cleanse. Thank you for sharing your stories and opening up your hearts. Thank you to all my wonderful patients. You are my treasures. I am honored for the opportunity to do life with you. You inspire me every day and you allow me to do what I love, Chiropractic.

Last but not least, "my boys." To my beloved husband, Mac, thank you for giving me the space and grace to write these words and follow my passion. To my son, Michael, thank you for letting "mom" write when I needed to. Thank you boys for all your unconditional love and support. You are God's greatest gift in my life.

> "Lord, Your discipline is good, for it leads to life and health. You restore my health and allow me to live!"
>
> —Isaiah 38:16

Contents

Acknowledgements xiii

Introduction 1

My Why 3

The Need to Detox 5

The Program 7

Detox Day 1: Getting Started 11

Detox Day 2: Be Prepared 15

Detox Day 3: Learning to Listen 19

Detox Day 4: Restoration 23

Detox Day 5: Grace 27

Detox Day 6: Stay on Track 33

Detox Day 7: Temptation 39

Detox Day 8: Pamper Yourself 45

Detox Day 9: Rejoice 49

Detox Day 10: Halftime 53

Detox Day 11: The Extra Mile 59

Detox Day 12: Holidays 63

Detox Day 13: Setbacks 69

Detox Day 14: It's Not Over 73

Detox Day 15: Re:Evaluate 77

Detox Day 16: Give Thanks 83

Detox Day 17: Choices 87

Detox Day 18: Rise 91
Detox Day 19: I Want Cake 95
Detox Day 20: Friendship 99
Detox Day 21: Building Blocks 103
The New Normal 107
Appendix A 109
Appendix B 113
Appendix C 117
About the Author 121
Notes 123

Introduction

Welcome to 21 days to a healthier you! As we get started, I want to encourage you to focus on the Big Picture, which is improved health. This Detox is truly about giving your body a rest from foods that overwork your digestive tract. It will also give your metabolism a boost and will teach you how to fuel your body properly. It's like the engine to a car. When you put the right fuel into your car, the performance is always better.

Remember, just as Rome was not built in a day, your unhealthy habits (or body) were not either. This program is not a quick easy weight loss diet. It is a jumpstart to a healthier you. Cleansing is a process and will take time, on your part, for success.

Over the next 21 days, you will learn how to give your body the nutrition it needs to function properly and efficiently. You will learn what influences may have led to your unhealthy lifestyle. There may be things about yourself you have forgotten or ignored or were too painful to deal with. I encourage you to look at everything that comes up for you. It might be like an onion, peeling back the layers from the inside out. The goal is to deal with it, learn from it, and let it go. Whether it is certain foods or habits or unhealthy thinking, let go of everything that is of no benefit to you and your body. It's time to learn new healthy habits and embrace a new you.

After the 21 days, you may discover you don't like coffee anymore or that you need to let go of dairy or choose less sugar in your diet. All in all, I am excited you are ready to make some serious changes in your health.

If you have never done a cleanse in your life, I am so glad you have enough courage to do this. It is definitely time! Once you have completed your first cleanse and detox, you will start to crave them more during the year. If you are facing a health challenge, a new illness, or diagnosis, this is a perfect start to reclaiming your health; however, make sure you give yourself grace. This is not about adding stress to your life. This cleanse is about getting your body cleaned out and ready to fight, ready to heal. Your body was MADE TO HEAL; it just needs a healthy environment to do so. It all starts here!

My Why

My life was forever changed, in 2010, when I was confronted with a health wake up call. My weight was at a record high and I was in no way taking care of myself. I was overworked, overstressed, and out of balance. I was in a total survival mode living off of sugar and caffeine to make it through my day. There is little wonder as to why I was in a health crisis. Actually, now, I call it my health opportunity because it was the jolt I needed to get my health back.

I CHANGED my lifestyle to eating a plant-based diet and giving my body the nutrition it desperately needed. I lost 46 pounds and my body was able to heal from my health opportunity.

Since then, I have been able to keep the weight off by maintaining many of the changes I am asking of you in this detox program. I am not claiming to be perfect, nor do I claim to have this all figured out. I have struggled with food my entire life. This is my reason for writing this book. Who better to help you than someone who can sit with you in the trenches and encourage you to be SUCCESSFUL. With everything in me, it is my passion to help you turn your HEALTH and LIFE around before it's too late. I am here to mentor you and coach you.

If you have a new health challenge, this is your wake up call. It's time to get busy. Make a choice to THRIVE and not just survive anymore.

What is your "WHY" for this cleanse?

The Need to Detox

A colleague of mine had a patient whose cholesterol was 344, triglycerides were 787, and heart risk was 7.2. AFTER the 21 days, she retook her blood test and her cholesterol was lowered to 187, triglycerides were 108, and her new heart risk was 3.7. Your body was made to heal! You just need to give it what it needs.

Before starting any program it is always important to share it with your healthcare professional. All the supplements are vegetarian and plant based, so there should be no side effects if you are taking medication.

I recommend getting lab work done before you start the 21 days so you can see the benefit to your health and share your results. Some basic blood tests you could request from your doctor are a Blood Glucose, Cholesterol, Triglycerides, and your CRP (C-Reactive Protein). CRP shows you if you have inflammation in your body.

Chronic inflammation is important to detect. If inflamation is present, it can mark the beginning of the gradual degeneration of an organ. Here are some of the diseases that such a sequence can cause:

Chronic Allergies

Jaundice

Kidney Disease

Acne

Hepatitis

Psoriasis

Blinding Headaches

AIDS

Arthritis

Pancreatitis

Chronic Fatigue Syndrome

Depression

Infections

Fibromyalgia

Septicemia

Multiple Joint Pain Syndrome

Dermatitis

Autoimmune Disorders

Candida Albicans

Cancer[1]

Startling, I know. Did you know that, "Scientists estimate that everyone alive today carries within her or his body at least 700 different toxins."[2] The Environmental Working Group has resource after resource to share with you the toxins we are exposed to every day. These toxins, over time, can wreak havoc on the body and promote disease and dysfunction.[3]

A noted surgeon, Dr. Harvey Kellogg, of the Kellogg Sanitarium in Battle Creek Michigan, spent most of his career studying the colons of living subjects. Kellogg is quoted as saying, "Of the 22,000 operations that I have personally performed, I have never found a single normal colon. Of the 100,000 that were performed under my jurisdiction, not over 6% were normal." Dr. Kellogg estimated that over 90% of the "diseases of civilization" were due to a blocked and non-functioning colon.[4]

Now if that is not motivation for you, I do not know what to say.

The Program

Here is the skinny. There are many detoxifying systems out there and on the market. Patients and friends ask me all the time about different supplements. My favorite one happens to be from Standard Process, a company that is the cleanest and most whole-food supplement company I know. In addition, they have been around for over 84 years. They have many research articles and awards you can review online at Standardprocess.com. Products are only available by a healthcare professional to make sure you receive the right nutrition for your body.

Your first option is to use the supplements and their clean, dairy-free protein powder to assist you on your cleanse. The second option is to just use the food and the protein powder in the program and not use the supplements. For the food only folks, I do recommend two shots of wheat grass per day for a minimum of eight days—one first thing in the morning and another before 3-4 p.m. (in case it gives you an energy jolt that lasts too long). If you do not have access to fresh wheat grass juice, you can use Evergreen. They are a company that has wheat grass flash frozen and it tastes good. Either way is a good start, but the supplements will support your body more efficiently. It will make the cleanse easier and more successful.

Regardless, the goal is NO Dairy, NO caffeine, NO sugar, and NO meat. Replaced with lots of water, fruit, vegetables, lentils, brown rice, and whey protein or rice protein.

(See Appendix B for The Battle Plan.)

AUTHORIZED FOOD LIST

The goal is to eat twice the amount of veggies as fruit. Think anything green and raw. Kale, collard greens, spinach, mustard greens, and red/green leaf lettuce are all great super-foods. If you steam your vegetables, make sure it is only for a few minutes. You may feel like there are too many restrictions and worry that you will be hungry the whole time; however, you will be surprised at how full you will be on this cleanse!

(For a more detailed list, see Appendix A.)

Vegetables:
(Organic when possible)

All vegetables

Fruits:
(Organic when possible)

Berries are lower in sugar, but there are no restrictions here. Just make sure your serving size is accurate for one. For example, bananas are high in sugar, so only use ½ of a banana. Go shopping and have fun! Whatever is in season and organic is the best!

Oils:

Coconut oil, Flax oil (Unheated), Olive oil (Extra-virgin), and Grapeseed oil

Sweeteners:

None, but if needed, date sugar and coconut sugar are low on the glycemic index.

AVOID

caffeine, sugar, alcohol, dairy, nuts/seeds, processed foods, and grains (except for wild or brown rice)

The goal is to have 2-3 protein shakes a day for the next 10 days. On Day 11, you can add fish and lean, clean protein (organic, grass-fed, no antibiotic meat). I recommend wild caught fish before the lean meat.

Make sure you prepare and do your grocery shopping first. Get your meals written down and a plan of attack ready. If you have any questions before starting, you can contact me through my website, www.madetoheal.com.

Top Three Things to Start:

1. Get your Meals Planned
2. Get your Groceries
3. Get your Goals

EXERCISE

This is a cleansing process. The only exercise you should be doing is light to moderate activity. Activities that will assist in the cleansing are walking, yoga, saunas, and massage. Walking truly is the best exercise right now. You can hit the gym later when this is over. The exercise will help increase circulation and assist you in removing toxins that may be held up in different organs of the body. I recommend doing a 20-30 minute walk a day. If you shoot for seven days you will end up walking for five days. Sometimes a nice walk will move toxins out and you will actually reveal some of your symptoms.

Note: You may find that your body needs more rest during the cleanse and that is okay! Listen to your body. It will tell you what it needs.

THE PERSONAL GUIDE

Just ahead you will find the first of twenty-two special daily messages, prepared just for you, to help you on this journey. I encourage you to stay right where you are and do not read ahead. It will be like Christmas every morning to see what special WORD or present was chosen for that day. I can hardly wait to hear all about your experiences and lifestyle changes and the positive impact the cleanse has had on your health. I'm excited to meet the NEW healthier you and it's just 21 days away!

Here's what a friend had to say about the messages, "I looked forward to your emails. They were informative, inspiring, and just the cheerleader that I needed. Knowing that there were other women going through it too was a big source of support. And having my husband be supportive was very helpful and encouraging."

This brings me to my next suggestion. Make sure you have a buddy or a group you can venture through this with. It will be more fun and you can share recipe ideas. Having that accountability partner will really help your success.

Have fun! You can do this!

DAY 1

Getting Started

Happy Day 1! I hope you are enjoying your morning and are eager to get started. I like to prepare for day one by taking the Gastro-Fiber the night before, on an empty stomach, just to get my body moving. Then, I start my first day with a tall glass of water and my first round of the cleanse. Then, I wait 20-30 minutes before I have my protein shake. If you are in a hurry, you can take the Gastro-Fiber with the smoothie.

The key is to send the supplements and food down your stomach and through your colon with great timing. It takes liquids and supplements 20-30 minutes to transition out of your stomach. Fruits and veggies take one to three hours transition time. Smoothies will take about an hour. The transition times will help you keep a smooth flow of easy things for your body to work on each day.

I am excited for you! Remember each day will build on the previous day. Make sure you journal during this time. As you release toxins, you also release emotions that are hanging out in the body. Let it all flow, then let it all go!

I want to encourage you to ask a few folks to be dedicated to praying for you over the next 21 days!

Today's Scripture:

> "Even strong young lions sometimes go hungry, but those who trust in the Lord will lack no good thing"
>
> —Psalm 34:10 [niv]

Enjoy your day!! Keep your water intake very high as you get started today. I love and appreciate you all!

Let's Pray

Heavenly Father,

I just want to thank You for my friend, who has been courageous enough to take on this 21-day cleanse. I pray for strength, endurance, and clarity over the next few weeks. Lord, please cover them from the top of their head to souls of their feet with your mercy and grace. I pray Your love surpasses all understanding in their encounters this week. I pray that this cleanse is the beginning of something fresh and new in their life! In Jesus' name, we pray, Amen.

Lessons Learned Today:

What was your success or win of the day?

____

____

____

____

What did you miss or misunderstand?

____

____

____

____

What is your goal for tomorrow?

What challenges came up today emotionally, spiritually or physically?

Journal Time:

Write a love note to yourself? Tell yourself you are worth the effort and time for this cleanse. You are beautifully and wonderfully made. You have a purpose beyond your imagination.

DAY 2

Be Prepared

Day one is under your belt! Congratulations! That is truly something to celebrate. By now, you probably have figured out what you can and cannot eat and have made your meal plan. On my day one, I enjoyed a delicious dinner of sautéed mushrooms, onions, garlic, and broccoli with liquid aminos (A healthy alternative to soy sauce, check it out). I combined the leftover lentils from lunch and BAM! Dinner! My husband loved it!

As you go through this process you will discover that the realities of detox can blind-side you. One day, while standing in line at a local craft store, I realized I was surrounded by every version of chocolate that was out for the holiday. Wow, it was an intense moment! I am glad to report that I made it just fine, but it was a challenge. That is why today's advice is: Be Prepared. Make sure you keep your snacks on you and ready.

Another time, I was shopping in the health food store when I could feel my blood sugar drop. These are the moments when you can easily break your detox by eating something off the menu. PREPARED equals SUCCESS! I was able to purchase some fruit and make it home, on track. I blended up a protein shake and felt my strength come back.

Today's Scripture

(This happens to be my LIFE verse. I hope it helps you!)

> "Lord, Your discipline is good, for it leads to life and health. You restore my health and allow me to live!"
>
> —Isaiah 38:16

Prepare for your day! Make two smoothies and take the second one to work or the office.

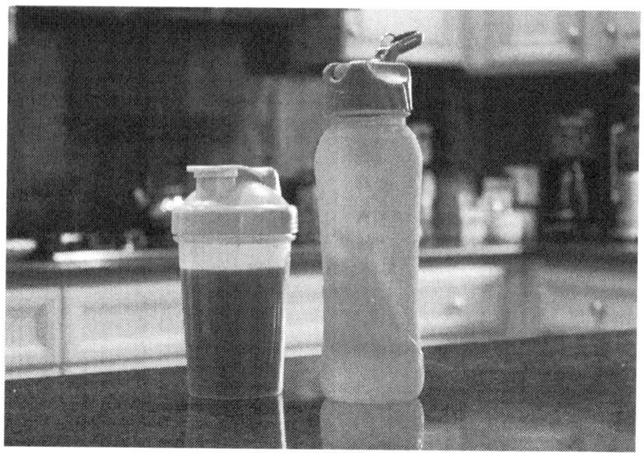

Let's Pray:

Heavenly Father,

Thank You for Your discipline. Thank you for this time of detoxifying our bodies to create space for healing in our lives, both emotionally and physically. Lord, I thank You for everyone who may read these words. May it encourage them whether they are on the program or not. Help us to commit this day to YOU! Show us when we need to surrender and give things to You completely! I pray for a successful, smooth day. I pray for clarity, rest, and rejuvenation. In Jesus' precious name, Amen.

Lessons Learned Today:

What was your success or win today?

____

____

____

____

What did you miss or misunderstand?

____

____

____

____

What challenges presented themselves today?

____

____

____

____

What are your goals for tomorrow?

____

____

____

____

Journal Time:

Take time to write what you are thankful for right now.

DAY 3

Learning to Listen

The Big Day 3 on any detox is usually a feeling of breakthrough. Your body has finally had a chance to adapt to the changes you presented it. No sugar, no caffeine, no meat, etc. The headaches should start to subside and the clarity will start to appear. Some normal detoxing symptoms may include bloating, unclear thinking, mild depression, aching in joints, flu-like symptoms, fatigue, headaches, itchy or irritated skin, increased bowel movements, or even constipation. There are some great herbal teas to help move things along. Also, make sure you are drinking plenty of water. I am talking 50-60 oz. a day, minimum (take your weight and divide by 2 = number of ounces of water per day). If this is your first detox ever, the headaches may last longer for you. I want to encourage you to press on! Make sure you are getting enough rest and the symptoms should lift.

Listen to your body. Only you know what your body needs as you are cleaning out toxins. For me, day three meant sleeping an extra hour. I missed my 5 a.m. wake up call, but I knew my body needed that extra hour of sleep. So, be flexible this week. Give yourself and your body grace. A few days of healthy cleansing food will result in positive life changes.

Today's Scripture:

> "Commit your actions to the Lord, and your plans will succeed."
>
> —Proverbs 16:3

Give the Lord this detox as a spiritual fast and see what He can do. We talked about changes in blood pressure, cholesterol, weight, allergies, low libido, and other toxic symptoms. These are your why and Jesus is your how.

Let's Pray:

Heavenly Father,

Thank You for this beautiful day. Thank You for our amazing bodies that you created. Thank you for allowing them the ability to heal from the inside out. Help us to listen to our bodies today and give them what they need. Maybe we need extra time, water, a walk, or a protein shake. Help us to stay committed to our plans so we can be successful and healthy. I pray for my friends walking through their busy days at work. I pray for Your favor in their day and help make things just a bit easier. In Jesus' precious name, Amen.

Lessons Learned Today:

What are you learning about yourself on this cleanse?

____

____

____

____

____

____

____

What keeps coming up for you as a struggle?

____

____

____

____

What's your commitment over the next few days?

____

____

____

____

Journal Time:

Think about what your body is trying to tell you and what God might be saying through that. Write down what messages are coming to you through this cleanse as you learn how to listen to your body and to God.

____

____

____

____

____

____

____

DAY 4

Restoration

I hope your days are getting easier on this program. My Day 4 provided me with some challenges. I made it through by following the program, even on a date with my beloved husband. I was so excited to see that the restaurant was serving Lentil soup! What a blessing that was!

Today, I want to focus on the restoration that is going on in your body. Focus on your Why for doing the cleanse. I don't know about you, but my pee has never been so clear, nor so frequent! That means your kidneys are healing and cleansing any impurities. Now, let's focus on your liver. It is becoming less clogged as you give it a break from fatty foods. Let's visualize our colons becoming radiant, free from disease and dysfunction. Today, call on the Lord for strength and confidence in getting this program done. Why? Because what you do today for your health will affect how your body works in 5, 10, or even 15 years from now.

My new find has been these dessert teas by The Republic of Tea. My friend Tawny, at the Healing Heart Vitamin store here in Moorpark, recommended them. They are delicious! I bought Red Velvet Chocolate and Chocolate Mint. They are such a great "treat" while still being legal on our program. Caffeine-free tea! For those of you missing the salty crunch taste, try some raw sun-dried tomato dehydrated chips. It is a raw tomato in a chip form. Gotta love the choices we have. (Please note: this is only to keep you on track. You will need to significantly increase your water consumption if you eat dehydrated food).

Today's Scripture:

> "'I will give you back your health and heal your wounds,' says the Lord."
>
> —Jeremiah 30:17

Our God is a God of restoration and healing!

Let's Pray:

Gracious Heavenly Father,

I pray, today, that Your mighty hand will be on the lives of those who have committed to this cleanse. I pray, also, for their families to see and experience the positive affects of this cleanse on their loved one. May they continue to grow in You during this cleanse and draw on YOUR STRENGTH when they need it. I pray for new healthy bodies from the inside outside. I pray for new lab results that require less medication. I pray for awesome testimonies of healing to share at the end of this program. Lord, I thank You for all You have done in my life and the lives of my friends. In Jesus' name we pray, Amen.

Lessons Learned Today:

What has God shown you today during this cleanse?

____

____

____

____

____

What has been your biggest breakthrough so far?

____

____

____

____

____

____

What was your success or win of the day?

____

____

____

____

____

____

What is your goal for tomorrow?

____

____

____

____

____

____

Remember-baby steps! Each day builds on the previous. Focus on how great you are going to feel at the end of the week.

Journal Time:

What seems to be on your heart today?

Surrender it, give it to God!

DAY 5
Grace

Today is a NEW day. The big day 5! I am so glad you have committed to this program. But here's the reality! You have to give yourself GRACE and say to yourself, "Way to go!" You are not going to be perfect. I want you to look at the big picture, especially, if this is your first detox program. Where you are now is better than it was five days ago. Where you are going to be in 5 or 16 more days will be increasingly better too. Give it your best effort. I know some of you are shocked by how well you are doing. Some of you may still be battling hunger and may need to make adjustments. That is totally okay! Look at what you have accomplished so far! No caffeine, no dairy, no meat, no carbs. You have replaced all those things with fruits, veggies, and so much more—a healthier you!

I have to share with you the experience a friend of mine had on the program. She had done everything "perfectly"—all the supplements, all the veggies, all the protein shakes—she really rocked it. Well, you know what, she ate half a bagel a few days into the program and she said it was like heaven. Did she go to detox jail? NO! She moves her body eight to nine hours a day with her job in physical fitness. She ate the bagel and she moved on! She refocused on the program. She considered all the good choices and changes she had made and then she had this Aha!! moment: "Wow, I really can add more veggies in my day after this program is over." She also commented on how much easier the shakes were getting and she was becoming quite creative with them. They were getting so good that her kids were stealing them from her. What a great example of giving yourself

GRACE. I want you to focus on the 80 or 99% good you have done and please do not condemn yourself for the unauthorized food bite that may have hit your lips.

I am so excited you have joined me on this adventure. I pray the next five days are going to show you the new changes you want to make in your life. Give yourself grace, but stay focused. And please, do not stress out about this process. You are doing so much better than you think.

Today's Scripture:

> "The Lord said, 'My Grace is all you need. My power works best in weakness.' So now I am glad to boast about my weaknesses, so that the power of Christ can work through me. That's why I take pleasure in my weaknesses, and in the insults, hardships, persecutions, and troubles that I suffer for Christ. For when I am weak, then I am strong."
>
> —2 Corinthians 12:9-10

I hope this encourages you today!

Let's Pray:

Gracious Heavenly Father,

Thank You so much for all You have taught us this week. Thank You for being our strength in our weakness. Lord, I ask You to give us supernatural strength today in all that we do. Whether we are cleaning our houses, making dinner for our family, or working on things for our jobs, Lord, I just ask You to shine through us today, knowing we have You in our lives. Show us any adjustments we need to make with our diet today. Help us to make this the most productive detox time ever! In Jesus' name, Amen.

I hope you have an awesome day . . . keep me posted on anything that comes up.

Lessons Learned Today:

What can you put on the grace table today?

____

____

____

____

____

What are you going to do better tomorrow?

____

____

____

____

____

What is better about your body today?

____

____

____

____

____

Are there any Aha!! moments you can speak about so far on your cleanse?

Remember the BIG picture! What is your Why?

Journal Time:

What other thoughts are on your heart today?

"Life and health are both simple when you go to the cause."

—Dr. Danita Thomas Heagy

DAY 6

Stay on track

Can you believe it has been six days?! I started getting comfortable about this time, which could be a good thing; however, I almost got derailed. I was with a friend who was helping me update my professional portrait to give me some new options. It was an all-day adventure (since it takes a village to get me dressed). It was a totally fun day; but, by 4 p.m., I was hungry. I mean really hungry.

Thankfully, we were in Malibu and decided to stop and have green smoothies on the way home. We found this great health food store. I was walking the aisles to find my son a snack and saw all these things I wanted to eat, but knew I shouldn't. Thankfully, my green smoothie came to the rescue! Ironically it was called "The Hulk!" Kale never tasted to good! It had kale, almond butter, almond milk, and a dash of cinnamon. It was AMAZING!! I kept thinking it tasted too good to be legal. But, thankfully, it was!

So, if this happens to you and you're almost ready to say forget it and just eat whatever . . . get back on TRACK! Stay the course! You are almost there.

Have you noticed there are so many healthy alternatives to foods you really enjoy? Tawny shared her recipe for raw, organic chocolate truffles, which are amazing. They provide a healthy alternative to chocolate; yet, it won't wreak havoc in the body. This recipe and a few more are in the Appendix.

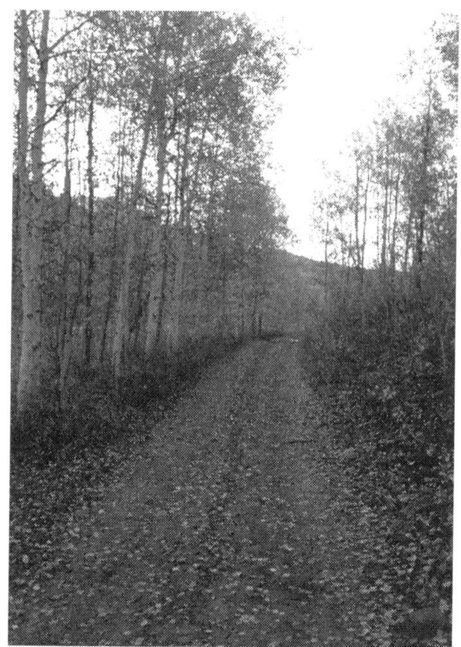

Today's Scripture:

"Trust in the Lord with all your heart and lean not on your own understanding; in all your ways acknowledge Him and He will make your paths straight."

—Proverbs 3:6

Let's Pray:

Lord,

Help us to stay on track today. Help us to keep You in our presence, moment by moment. Help us not to lean on our own strength, because many times we fail. I thank You and praise You for everyone who reads these words. I pray for them and their family. I pray for healing in their body and direction for the path they need to walk. We are all on different paths and journeys; yet, I am so grateful You know every step we take! I am humbled and grateful for this week. I pray for those in our lives who are struggling with major illness or disease. Guide them on the path You want them to take, so they may be healed and healthy again. In Jesus precious name, Amen!

Have a blessed day ladies and gentlemen! Send me your funny stories or Aha!! moments. I would love to share in those moments with you.

Lessons Learned Today:

What was your success or win today?

____

____

____

____

____

____

What helped you through your day that you didn't expect?

____

____

____

____

____

What challenges came up today?

____

____

____

____

____

What are your goals for tomorrow?

____

____

____

____

____

____

____

Remember:

> "You never know how far reaching what you may say, think, or do today will affect the lives of millions tomorrow."
>
> —BJ Palmer

Journal Time:

What can you do today that will bless others tomorrow?

____

____

____

DAY 7

Temptation

I love receiving emails and text messages with positive feedback of how people are doing on the program. I am truly excited for each and every one. I am so glad to share your joy as you reap the benefits of the cleanse—which is why we do this often. Many of you have lost five to six pounds, you are feeling less bloated, leaner, or you just feel great on the inside! My prayer for you is that you stay on this path as long as possible. The barrier to this, however, is that life and TEMPTATIONS love to get in the way.

Have you had temptations this week? Here is one that was sent to me during a previous detox! Look at what someone said NO to! I am so proud of her! I might have eaten the cherry for sure!

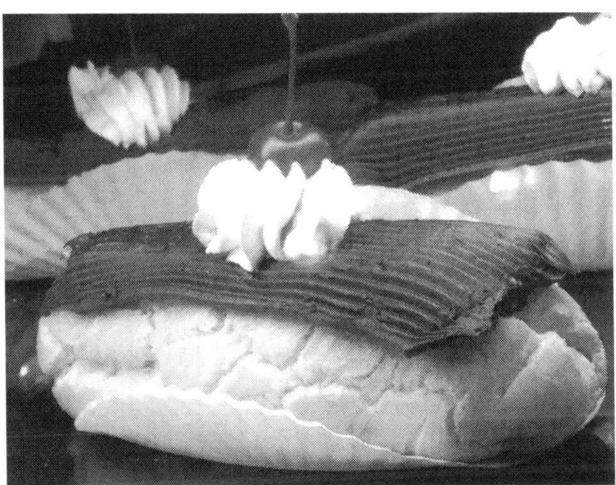

I had the pleasure of making two dozen cupcakes for my son's class. Talk about temptation! For the first time EVER in

MY LIFE, I did not eat one cupcake! I tasted the batter to make sure it mixed well, but not enough to throw me off the detox program. I was so happy. For that moment, I didn't even want them. The focus and the hard work during the first seven days of detox was in full effect. I have to share with you that this has never happened. I usually eat a few cupcakes and any leftover frosting! Not this time, friends. I finished icing the cupcakes and strategically put the icing containers in the trash bins outside, leaving no room for temptation!

So, how do you handle your temptations? Do you walk away, pray, or maybe just take a bite? Whatever your strategy, there is such JOY when you overcome the temptation. I know it's difficult at that moment, so, change your environment if you can. If you can wait for ten minutes, your brain can usually reset its focus. I also take the Gymnema herb (you should have some in your kit) which helps curb cravings. It really works!

I am so thankful for you; and, although I am not with you, I want you to know that I am here for you. I am cheering you through the words in this book. I pray continuously that every person who takes part in this cleanse will be blessed. You are not doing this alone. Why is this important? Because there is power in numbers and in prayer. I truly believe there is strength in accountability; otherwise, I would never have made it through 24 cupcakes! Whoo Hoo! If it was just me doing the cleanse, I would have said, "Oh who cares, it's just one." So make sure you have a buddy and/or me to check in with. It makes it more fun when you share your successes or even your moments of oops.

Today's Scripture:

> "Don't tear apart the work of God over what you eat. Remember, all foods are acceptable, but it is wrong to eat something if it makes another person stumble. It is

> better not to eat meat or drink wine or do anything else if it might cause another believer to stumble."
>
> —Romans 14:20-21

I know God is working in you this week. He is busy healing your body, your mind and spirit. So, I encourage to you to keep up the great work and may this verse be food for your soul. I love and appreciate you so much.

Let's Pray:

> Heavenly Father,
>
> Thank You so much for all that You do for us. Even the little things we may not notice in our day. Lord, help us with our temptations today. Help us to recognize them and give them to You completely! We know by Your power and strength, we can do all things! We love and appreciate You, Lord. Thank You for walking with us through this cleanse. Give us a deeper understanding of our body and our health. In Jesus' name we pray, Amen!

Thank you, friends, for making it a full week! The hardest part is over, so, I know you can do another week. What's one more week out of the fifty-two, right?! I know you can do it! I am praying for you!

Lessons Learned Today:

What was or has been your temptation in life?

____

____

____

What was your win or success today?

____

____

____

____

What do you need to write off and start fresh tomorrow?

____

____

____

____

____

What are your goals for tomorrow?

____

____

____

____

____

Journal Time:

Write a note to your temptations. Tell them they have no more power over you. Tell them they do not serve you nor your body. Tell them to get lost, right now, in the name of Jesus!

____

____

TEMPTATION

DAY 8

Pamper Yourself

It's the home stretch of the first phase of detox. Things should be getting easier and boring at the same time. Your goal today is to pamper yourself. Do something special for yourself. I like to schedule a massage and a facial for my pamper days. Yes, I love getting spoiled! However, if I don't plan it, it will never happen! All you have is today, so find ways to make it outstanding!

If you want to plan a special treat, here are some healthy ways to pamper yourself yet curb sugar cravings. These tips will work now and after the detox, so you can maintain all your hard work.

1. Raw chocolate – high in antioxidants and lower in sugar (after detox)
2. Almond Butter, Cacao Truffles
3. Teeccino – herbal coffee and that brews up like a tea. Many flavors including Chocolate, Vanilla Nut, Hazelnut, and Chocolate Mint.
4. Dessert Teas – Republic of Tea has some wonderful scrumptious flavors of tea. They are very warm and comforting without any calories or sugar effects on the body.
5. Spoonful of Raw Cacao Nibs and Almond Butter.

Today's Scripture:

"Don't you realize that your body is the temple of the Holy Spirit, who lives in you and was given to you by God?"

—1 Corinthians 6:19

So today, go for a hike, a walk with a friend, sit in the park for a bit. Do something different and take a moment to reflect on all that has happened this week.

Let's Pray:

Dear Lord,

Help my friends make themselves a priority in their day. Help them not to schedule every single hour of the day away. Meet us where we need You Lord, right in the sweet or hard place in our heart. Show us what we can do to make our hearts sing. In Jesus' name, Amen.

Reminder: Start taking the Green Food supplement. You no longer need to take the Cleanse supplement. If you are on the Food-Only path, you can continue with wheat grass shots or taper off to one a day. The benefits of wheat grass out weigh any dosage. So, be encouraged to continue if you can for the next 21 days.

Lessons Learned Today:

What did you do today to pamper yourself?

____

____

____

____

What are you grateful for today?

____

____

____

____

____

What was the one thing you did great today?

____

____

____

____

____

What are you willing to add into your daily routine after the cleanse?

____

____

____

____

____

What are your goals for tomorrow?

____

____

____

____

____

Journal Time:

Write about how difficult or easy it is to pamper yourself. Do you struggle with making yourself a priority? If yes, why? What can you do to put yourself on the list?

"And may you have the power to understand, as all God's people should, how wide, how long, how high, and how deep His love is." (For YOU!)

—Ephesians 3:17-19

DAY 9

Rejoice

Good Morning this fine morning of Day 9. How are you feeling? The word REJOICE feels right for Day 9. REJOICE that you have done so well on this detox. REJOICE in how amazing you feel. I pray you continue to do well and feel amazing.

Remember, yesterday you were to start using the Green Food supplement which is packed with kale, broccoli sprouts, and alfalfa sprouts. These are Superfoods that prevent cancer and heal your colon. If you forgot, that's okay, just start today. You no longer need to take the cleanse. Just add the Green Food and continue with the Gastro-Fiber. Make adjustments for your body if you need to. Maybe take the Gastro-Fiber twice a day, if needed.

You have one more official day on Phase I. Then, on day 11, you get to add some clean fish or lean meat, such as chicken. You can continue the protein shakes and take the Green Food. I am excited for you! Are you staying focused?

If you are done with the word "Detox," I want you to think of this as your "NEW NORMAL." You don't necessarily have to detox to keep on a healthy track. Maybe you keep the protein shakes in your life and you keep adding more fresh fruits and veggies. I recommend you continue the Green Food just as a great prevention of any illness. Lots to think about, but, today, LET's Rejoice!

Today's Scripture(s):

"No wonder my heart is glad, and I rejoice. My body rests in safety."

—Psalm 16:9

"This is the day that the Lord has made. We will rejoice and be glad in it."

—Psalm 118:24 [nkjv]

Let's Pray:

Dear Lord,

Thank You so much for this day. Thank You for helping us with our detox over the last nine days. I am so grateful for the changes our bodies have made. Give each person the feeling of rest and peace in their bodies. I pray that this would encourage more friends and family members to try a detox program for the first time. Lord, bless our day as we REJOICE in You and our success of the last week. In Jesus' name, Amen.

Friends, have a blessed day! Share with me your successes, breakthroughs, or Aha!!! moments. You may be able to help someone as I share them with other groups.

Lessons Learned Today:

What can you REJOICE about today?

____

____

____

____

____

____

____

What is better about your body that you have noticed?

____

____

____

____

____

____

____

What has this cleanse inspired you to do in the future?

____

____

____

____

____

____

____

What would you share with someone who is just starting out on Day 1?

____

____

____

____

____

Journal Time:

Write down and share what you are so thankful for? What can you rejoice about and tell others?

DAY 10

Halftime

You made it! 10 days with NO dairy, NO caffeine, NO sugar, NO meat; just fruit, veggies, salads, brown rice, and lentils. Just as with any race, once you get through it, you say to yourself, "I can do that again." Or "I want to do another one." I hope for the first-timers in the detox world, it was not as scary as you anticipated. I hope you noticed some amazing differences in your body over the last week. You should notice more energy, more clarity, less bloating, inches off your waist, or even 5-10 pounds of weight loss. These are all bonuses to the benefits you gave your body by cleansing from the inside out. You gave your kidneys and liver a break from major work. It was like they took a vacation and now they are supercharged and ready to get back to work keeping you healthy.

Here's your next challenge: ten days of phase II of the detox program. Everything you did, plus, more protein at lunch and dinner. I recommend sticking to wild caught, clean fish. If you need to add some free range, organic clean chicken a few times in the next week, that is okay. Do your best to avoid feeling deprived. Have a bite of something you've been missing or make the raw chocolate truffles to stay the course. Whatever you choose, you are awesome! I am so proud of you and all the hard work you have done.

Now, you get to add a little more protein to help keep you going. This is a healthy way to lose one to two pounds of weight a week and keep it off—permanently. Remember, it takes 21 days to develop a new habit. I look forward to hearing all the new changes you have implemented into your life.

I want to close again with my life verse. It is so perfect right now. You have detoxed your body from all the old unhealthy habits. Detoxing feels disciplined and structured, yet leaves you feeling so super charged. Eating like this is how my body runs best. The key is not letting emotional eating wiggle its way back in. It's a spiritual war and I want us to win.

Today's Scripture:

> "Lord, Your disciple is good, for it leads to life and health. You restore my health and allow me to live!"
>
> —Isaiah 39:16

Let's stay here friends, restored, healthy and able to live the life God intended!

Let's Pray:

Heavenly Father,

Thank You for this gift of awareness! The awareness of our body and how You intended for it to function. Help us to look at food as fuel and nothing else. Only You can heal the pain in our hearts. There truly is "no cookie big enough," you know I have tried looking! Father, help us to be empowered to challenge ourselves for another ten days for You. You have shown us so much more, help us to go the distance with something we have already started. We love You and praise You for all our successes so far. We want more breakthroughs and more lasting changes. So we surrender our old habits and we thank You for implementing new ones. Thank You for my friends across the country sharing in Your glorious changes. In Jesus' name, Amen.

Lessons Learned Today:

How are you doing? Really?

____

____

____

____

____

Are you feeling stronger and more clear?

____

____

____

____

____

The momentum really gets started here. It's halftime! Your body is going to start to enjoy the program and perform much better. What have you noticed so far?

____

____

____

Any struggles?

____

____

____

____

____

Are you committed to the second half?

____

____

____

____

____

I know you can do it! The hard part is over. Now, you get to eat lean protein and shift to the Green Food supplements.

Journal Time:

Take a breath. You can do this! I am with you all the way!

Write down your successes so far. How much weight have you lost, how many inches, what symptoms have been alleviated? Write down your goals for the second half.

____

____

____

DAY 11
The Extra Mile

Have you ever run a 5k or 10k, or played a sport where it took all you had to make it through the last mile or last quarter of the game? Well, instead of depleting your body and wearing it out, this EXTRA MILE is going to add years to your life. It will help your body heal. It may even reverse lifestyle diseases like high blood pressure, diabetes, or even high cholesterol.

I am so excited you are on board and part of this National Cleanse! I am praying for all the new ideas and things you are discovering in this book and in your groups at home. What you do today could inspire someone else to make big LIFE changes.

You have made it through the first ten days, now it's time to kick it up a notch! It's time to dig deep and see what God really wants to reveal to you. Maybe He wants you to continue making these new changes in your daily routine. Maybe He wants to heal you of some old wounds you keep stuffing with food. Whatever it is, it's time to dig deep and go the EXTRA MILE, for you and you alone. You are the only one responsible for your own health. Not your husband, your wife, your significant other, your mother, your father, your . . . whomever! Sweet friend, it's just you!

When I was lying face down for almost two hours getting a breast biopsy done, there wasn't anyone I could I blame, or complain to. It was me who chose to make unhealthy choices that landed me on that table.

That's why we have to go the EXTRA MILE, now! To prevent, to fight, to heal our bodies no matter what comes our way.

Today's Scripture:

"What, then, shall we say in response to these things? If God is for us, who can be against us?"

—Romans 8:31

Let's Pray:

Heavenly Father,

Thank You so much for all Your strength, Your power, and Your love. Help us to dig deep and go the extra mile in this cleanse. Show us, God, what we need to add to our lives and what we need to omit. We may already know the answer, but Lord give us the tools and pathway to make it happen, once and for all! I pray for my friend reading this right now. Meet them and comfort them right where they are. In Jesus' name, Amen.

Lessons Learned Today:

What does going the EXTRA MILE mean to you right now?

____

____

____

____

____

____

____

____

What do you think God is trying to reveal to you along this journey?

____

____

____

____

____

____

What do feel your biggest obstacle is right now?

____

____

____

____

____

____

How can someone help you remove or lighten that same obstacle?

____

____

____

____

____

Journal Time:

What emotions or thoughts are coming up for you today after reading this section?

> "I was always looking outside myself for strength and confidence but it comes from within. It is there all the time."
>
> —Anna Freud

DAY 12

Holidays

It's Halloween as I am writing this. The kick off to the holiday season! While I was purchasing the candy for my little visitors, the store was already putting up Christmas cards. That means it's time to get ready and dive in with a new perspective. If not, then it can become three months of careless choices resulting in 10-20 pounds of weight gain.

Here are some questions you can ask yourself as you face a holiday:

1. How will this candy or treat make me feel after I eat it?
2. What is the bigger effect on my body on the inside? Does it have GMOs? Is it organic?
3. Can I just enjoy this treat and move on? Or is this going to trigger more food?
4. What are my health goals right now? Is this going to help me or delay me?
5. Can I say NO and choose something better for me later?

Whether it's Halloween, a birthday party, or an anniversary, you are going to be faced with some difficult choices. There will always be temptations to trigger bad habits. The key is to be prepared! Make sure you eat your healthy meal at home before you go to parties. Drink a protein shake before you leave so you are not starving and can stay in control. Have a quick snack in your purse or the car to keep you on track. This is a great time to try out some of those delicious alternative recipes from the appendix.

Now, today, if you just lose it and eat the junk, just count it as a vegetable and move on! Get back on your detox program tomorrow and stay the course. The goal here is making small LIFE changes. The other big goal is to LOVE yourself. Check in with your body and see what you need today. Make sure today is inspiring and empowering, NOT DEPRIVING!

I love and appreciate you all.

Today's Scripture:

> "This is My commandment: Love each other in the same way I have loved you."
>
> —John 15:12

I know it's easier for to LOVE others, but today LOVE yourself. Take a moment for yourself.

Let's Pray:

> Heavenly Father,
>
> We thank You so much for waking us up today. Thank You for giving us life and breath. Lord, I pray for a fun day with family and friends. Help us to take our focus off food and keep it on relationships with friends, spouses, colleagues, even our neighbors. Help us to walk in a place of gratitude and love wherever we go. I thank You for prayers that have been answered for those facing a health challenge. You are the Great Physician and we continue to pray for friends on our heart today. In Jesus' name, we pray, Amen.

It truly is an honor and a privilege to walk with you in this amazing journey called life!

Lessons Learned Today:

What holiday or event is coming your way?

____

____

____

____

____

____

What is your plan to be successful at the event?

____

____

____

____

____

____

What is your commitment to your cleanse right now?

____

____

____

____

____

What was your success or win today?

____

____

____

____

What's your motivation or Why for pressing on tomorrow?

____

____

____

____

What's your plan or goal for tomorrow?

____

____

____

____

____

Who can you enlist to help keep you accountable to your goals?

____

____

____

____

____

Journal Time:

Spend some time thinking about what the holidays mean to you—the events, the customs, the festive foods, and the comfort foods—and how you can still celebrate the meaning of those traditions while making healthy choices. Write out a plan for how to keep your holidays special while keeping on track with your new goals.

DAY 13

Setbacks

The word for today is SETBACKS. It has been thirteen days of following a really disciplined program and being focused. You may have experienced some setbacks, not just in your diet, but, in your body. Your body may be healing an old injury that happened a year ago or more. Or maybe you have had a day where you just want to take a time out and turn off the world.

The definition of setback is: "An unanticipated or sudden check in progress; a change from better to worse."[5] You see it's that unanticipated part that really drives me crazy. We have things to do, people to see and then our body "takes a sudden check in progress." Mine was my lower back. A year ago I really hurt it. I was laid out for six weeks and I could not see patients or do anything. My disc still gets inflamed from time to time, putting me in a "check in progress" mode. It can be so discouraging when we are forced to take an unexpected break. It really helps me relate and have compassion for my patients.

Today, if you are experiencing some of these setbacks in life, whether they are physical, or financial, or spiritual, remember, they are not forever. Let's call them hiccups or even speed bumps in the road. A place to get better from worse, a place to grow. All the good nutrition you have been fueling your body with has been healing it from the inside out. So remember, SETBACKS are not FOREVER, they are just HICCUPS.

Today's Scripture:

"Dear brothers and sisters, when troubles come your way, consider it an opportunity for great joy. For you know that when your faith is tested, your endurance has a chance to grow. So let it grow, for when your endurance is fully developed, you will be perfect and complete, needing nothing."

—James 1:1-4

Let's Pray:

Gracious Heavenly Father,

Thank You for our setbacks. The moments that keep us humble and not in complete control. We know You have everything under Your control! Help us to see our "checks in progress" as golden opportunities for growth and direction of the path You have us on. Help us to focus on You, Lord. Show us the directions we need to take just for today. Thank You for the wonderful treasures that are in my life, in my office and reading these words. Reach out and touch their hearts in a way only YOU know HOW. I pray for healing for everyone that this touches today. You are able to heal anyone You choose. I pray for faith, endurance and a supernatural strength. In Jesus' name, we pray . . . and everyone said, "Amen!"

Thanks for letting me share my heart. I hope it blesses you and encourages you.

Lessons Learned Today:

What setbacks are you facing right now?

____

____

What can you do to give yourself grace?

What are your goals for tomorrow?

What's your focus for the rest of the cleanse?

Journal Time:

What's on your heart, is there something frustrating you, write it all out?

DAY 14

It's Not Over

The day is not over! I hope you had a blessed day focused on your detox and making strides in creating a new you. Have you ever been jolted out of a good sleep? One morning I was jolted out of bed to move my car for the new street paving. It threw off my routine and I really missed my quiet time that morning. Thankfully, I was able to fit it in later that night.

To be honest, that whole day proved to be a challenge. I battled the pull toward sugar all day. But I stuck to the program and it really helped. I had lentils, brown rice, and fish for lunch. Can I get an AMEN for Whole Foods? Healthy, yummy prepared food ready to go. I also focused on my protein shakes and had some fruit for snacks. Not sure why I had the shift, but the cool thing was my awareness of it. I just took notice of it and let it flow. Can you relate?

Today's Scripture:

> "God is able to do more than we ask or think through His power working in us."
>
> —Ephesians 3:20

I am not sure how your day went, but I am thankful I can rest in God and all He is able to do. From healing to caring, He covers it all. I hope you can stand on this verse and give God all your cares tonight. He is ready for them so He can give you rest.

Let's Pray:

Heavenly Father,

Thank You for this cherished time! Thank You for the wonderful people I get to share and do life with. It truly is a blessing. I pray for rest tonight. I pray for Your Almighty Power to do something amazing in our hearts. Give us a peace, give us hope, and give us strength to do what You have called us to do. No matter how small or HOW BIG, give us the baby steps we need to walk in Your blessings. We thank You and praise You for everything. In Jesus' name we pray, Amen.

Lessons Learned Today:

What can I do to be better prepared for the curve balls life throws my way?

____

____

____

____

How can I be more attuned to the triggers that could derail my progress?

____

____

____

____

____

How can I take a lesson from these unexpected events and use them to help with my progress?

____

Journal Time:

List at least five lifestyle changes you think you will make after Day 21.

DAY 15
Re:Evaluate

Can you believe you have been eating this great for fifteen days? Is it starting to get contagious? Once you start feeling great and you slip up on an "unauthorized" food, you may surprise yourself as to how quickly you get back on your plan.

Today, I want you to reevaluate where you are. In chiropractic, we do re-exams to note our client's progress. It shows us what areas have improved and what areas we still need to work on. So here's a little checklist to see how you are doing:

1. Water: How's your water intake? The number of ounces should be equal to half your weight.
2. Protein Shakes: One to two per day. Going well?
3. Supplements: Super Green Food and Gastro-Fiber . . . still on track?
4. Meals: Good clean veggies, fruit (Snacks), clean meats
5. Balance: How's your balance with everything? Life, work, detox, exercise?

How did you do? I so hope you are doing great and moving forward. Each time you do a detox program, you get better and better at it. Sure, it might be challenging some days, but you are really taking your health to the next level when you detox your body. I know we are quick to look at where we are not perfect. I want you to focus on what you are doing well. Then, focus on one thing you can improve. Maybe, take your supplements with you so you do not forget. Or maybe plan your meals tonight for tomorrow, so you stay on track.

I attended a memorial service recently. They didn't share this person's mistakes in life. They shared how he blessed his family and helped others—from raising eleven children with his beautiful wife, to being the local plumber, or growing veggies in his garden. Life is a dash as you know it.

This reminded me of my call to help as many people as possible. Thank you for the opportunity to inspire you to be healthy and whole from the inside out.

Today's Scripture:

> "If your gift is serving others, serve them well. If you are a teacher, teach well. If your gift is to encourage others, be encouraging. If it is giving, give generously. If God has given you leadership ability, take the responsibility seriously. And if you have a gift for showing kindness to others, do it gladly."
>
> —Romans 12:7-8

Let's Pray:

Heavenly Father,

Thank You for my friends making it to DAY 15! On this day of reevaluation, show them adjustments they need to make to finish strong. Help them focus on their water, protein shakes and supplements. Guide them through any emotions that come up today. Make their day easy and light. In Jesus' name, Amen.

Lessons Learned Today:

How is my progress going?

____

____

____

____

____

____

____

What roadblocks have I encountered and how did I work around them?

____

____

____

____

____

What continues to be my biggest obstacle?

____

____

____

____

____

What keeps me motivated for moving forward?

Journal Time:

Write about what you are doing great so far on the cleanse followed by what needs a little more attention from your checklist.

Your checklist:

1. Water: How many ounces?

2. Protein shakes?

3. Supplements:

4. Meals

5. Balance: Life, work, family, etc.

Of the above list, make a note where you need to focus.

DAY 16

Give Thanks

Today let's just give thanks for all the blessings we have. From the pillow we get to lay our heads on at night to the family and friends who walk with us through life. Today, let's surrender any food issues, body issues, health issues, and life issues and just give them to God. All I know is God is able and greater than anything we can imagine. So, today, let's share all He has done in our lives. We have so much to be thankful for and God is worthy of our praise!

Today's Scripture:

> "I will give thanks to the Lord with all my heart. I will tell of all the great things You have done. I will be glad and full of joy because of YOU. I will sing praise to Your name, O Most High"
>
> —Psalm 9:1-2

> "I will speak with the voice of thanks, and tell of all Your great works."
>
> —Psalm 26:7

Let's Pray:

Gracious Heavenly Father,

Thank You for today. Thank You for all the gifts You have given us. Thank You for our children, our spouses, our family, and our friends. Thank You for providing for us and our every need. Thank You for our hearts to love one another as You have loved us. Thank You for our bodies. We ask that they would find complete healing with Your guidance. Thank You for this ministry you have given me. I pray that You bless all my friends today who read these words. Comfort them in their deepest places, so they know it could only be from YOU, Lord. In Jesus' name, Amen.

Lessons Learned Today:

What does gratitude really mean to me?

____

____

____

____

____

____

What am I most thankful for?

____

____

____

____

____

____

What challenge in my life can I try to see in a new way so I can also be grateful for it?

____

____

____

____

____

How does being grateful help me on my journey?

____

____

____

____

____

Journal Time:

Take out a sheet of paper and randomly write EVERYTHING you are thankful for! Be creative!

____

____

____

____

____

____

DAY 17

Choices

Only a few more days on this "cleanse," and I know you probably can't wait to get back to eating a little less restrictively. Remember, this is just for a moment and the goal is to look at making NEW CHOICES. It takes 21 days to develop a new habit, so I hope you are ready to add some new choices to your daily life.

Here's your homework! I want you to email your accountability partner three new choices you are going to make after the cleanse is over. This step is how I have made lasting changes over the past two years. Two years ago, I wrote down no carbonated drinks, no caffeine and no more meat. It was something on my heart I knew I could let go of in my life. What is in your life you noticed you could let go of in the last seventeen days?

In order for this to work, you have to write it down! Feel free to email me! I would love to hear from you about how this cleanse has helped you. If you share, you could be helping someone else take the first step to healthier life.

In my son's devotion one evening, we read about choices. "When your greatest desire is to please Me, making the right choices becomes easier. A quick, one-word prayer, 'Jesus' is all it takes to call upon My help and guidance. Seek to please Me in everything you do."[6]

Today's Scripture:

> "Take delight in the Lord, and He will give you your heart's desires."
>
> —Psalm 37:4

Let's Pray:

Dear Heavenly Father,

I pray that each person would call on Jesus today when they need to make hard choices or even the smallest of choices. Help them to know You are with them. In Jesus' name, Amen.

I hope you are inspired by your new choices that will change your health and your life! If you or a friend needs to chat, pray, or need some medical direction, I would love to help. Don't forget to email someone your top three choices!

Lessons Learned Today:

How do I really feel about accountability?

____

____

____

____

____

What is the most difficult choice I've faced during this cleanse?

____

____

____

____

____

What is the most difficult choice I've ever faced?

How did I handle each of those choices? Could I have made better ones? Did my experience affect how I made future choices?

Journal Time:

DAY 18

Rise

Good Morning! It's time to RISE and shine! Don't forget to email me the three things you are going to change after this cleanse. If you cannot think of three, give me one thing you are going to change.

As you know, diets do not work, but lifestyle changes do. In the book, Lose it For Life, the authors shares an acronym to help us take action to create a regular habit. It's called "RISE: Reduce, Increase, Substitute, and Eliminate.[7] Stephen Arterburn recommends this as an action formula for each area we need to change. Some days I feel like, "Give me chocolate or nothing else will do." Now, I can reduce the amount, increase the quality to raw chocolate, substitute it to cacao nibs or simply eliminate it. Certain days of the month I can eliminate chocolate, but some days a nice cup of hot cacao powder mixed with water does the trick. It's healthy, high in antioxidants, and no sugar! Bam! It's a great substitute without going crazy and feeling deprived.

I hope you are excited about all the healthy options available! They are free from all the genetically modified foods, preservatives and additives that are lethal to your body. Shop your local health food store and find substitutions for your favorite foods and even your body care products. It doesn't have to be expensive either. Shop around and you will find the best prices or even items on sale. You and your family are worth it!

> "God loves you just the way you are, but He refuses to leave you that way."[8]
>
> —Max Lucado

Let's RISE to the challenge and make ourselves better from the inside out! We were called to take great care of our bodies, like the temple or our house. I heard this my whole life, but I didn't make the shift until I had a health opportunity. Don't wait until you have a health opportunity. Make the changes now and prevent any health issues you can.

Today's Scripture:

> "Or didn't you realize that your body is a sacred place, the place of the Holy Spirit? Don't you see that you can't live however you please, squandering what God paid such a high price for? The physical part of you is not some piece of property belonging to the spiritual part of you. God owns the whole works. So let people see God in and through your body."
>
> —1 Corinthians 6:18-20 [msg]

Let's Pray:

Heavenly Father,

Thank You for my friend joining us on our detox journey. I pray that You would help us rise to changes you have whispered to us in our hearts. Help us to make lifestyle changes that will only glorify You in our bodies. Lord, You have given us life, hope, and a faith to conquer anything we desire. I pray that You show my friends what they need to do to conquer any challenges they may have. We give You this day. In Jesus' name, Amen.

Lessons Learned Today:

What three things do you think you could get rid of in your diet?

____

____

____

____

____

____

What do you think you could reduce in your diet?

____

____

____

____

____

What do you think you could substitute in your diet or maybe make into a healthier choice?

____

____

____

____

____

Journal Time:

How does R.I.S.E. speak to you? What do think you need to reduce, increase, substitute, or eliminate? Write what speaks to your heart.

"Our greatest glory is not in never failing, but in rising up every time we fail."[9]

—Ralph Waldo Emerson

DAY 19

I Want Cake

Really? I was almost done with my cleanse and my body started screaming, "I want cake!" Do I really need cake or just some time with Jesus? I was avoiding myself and this was a true indicator that I had to check in to see what was up! Have you ever sat yourself down in a quiet place to see what was really going on? Or do you keep yourself too busy and ignore what's really going on inside of you. I was tiptoeing into some old habits. You know those days you just want to check out of your life. I had no interest in getting things done or reflecting on what was really going on.

Today, I am going to share with you something I discovered. I kind of don't like myself sometimes. Have you ever had those days where you take care of everyone else in your day, but when it comes to you, you just let yourself go. I love taking care of people! It truly is my gift and calling. But, when it comes to time for ME, I fall short. Anyone relate?

One of my son's recent vocabulary words was worthy, "deserving of." We are children of the Most High God. We are royalty, so worthy of abundance and blessings beyond our imagination. Why do we get in the way of our success in health, relationships, and our finances? Not feeling worthy has shown up in my heart on many occasions. I need to recognize these feelings when they show up and get rid of them, forever. They don't serve me at all. How about you?

After reading and being in God's presence, all the worry and worthless seeds left my heart. I was finally able to shake the emotional drive toward a craving. I am not perfect, and I do not have it all together . . . at all! But I confess it and surrender it to God and I move on.

I am glad to report that instead of cake, I ate a RAW Revolution bar called "Chocolate Crave" and it was delicious. Other things you can do to take care of yourself are go for a walk, be outside in nature, read, write, have a chat with a friend, and hug someone you love.

Today's Scripture:

> "Then Jesus said to His disciples: Therefore, I tell you, do not worry about your life, what you will eat; or about your body, what you will wear."
>
> —Luke 12:22

Jesus wants to be with us and we need to practice being in the Peace of His Presence, along with, being present with ourselves. I hope this helps when you have a challenging day! I hope you feel good and back on track!

Let's Pray:

Heavenly Father,

Thank You for being with us even when we don't want to be in our own skin. Thank You for taking away our worry and our fears. You are a God able to move mountains and heal our hearts in a moment. I lift up anyone who is struggling today or this week. Comfort them and share with them how worthy and important they are to You. We are all Your children and we really do matter. Help us to understand this so we can create a life and the health You have called us to enjoy. In Jesus' name we pray, Amen!

Lessons Learned Today:

What has been your most challenging day?

____

____

____

____

What helped you get through your mountain of a day?

____

____

____

____

____

What new habits or things did you do to defuse that bomb?

____

____

____

____

What did you learn about yourself this time?

____

____

____

____

What are three things you might try when you are faced with another challenging day?

____

____

____

____

Journal Time:

Write about the last time you abandoned yourself or did not take care of yourself. You know, the time you should have said "No" to someone because you were exhausted. What situation comes to mind?

____

____

____

____

____

____

____

____

____

____

____

____

DAY 20
Friendship

Has someone ever hacked into your world? I had a little curve ball thrown my way through social media. Someone was sending crazy messages from my Twitter account. Not fun! All in all, I managed to navigate through the challenges and had the best day with my amazing practice members. They truly bless me and inspire me every day.

Today, the word that has been on my heart is "Friendship." Many of us are blessed with amazing friends and we take great care of those relationships. I know yesterday I shared about sometimes not "liking" myself. So, my goal today was to be "friends" with myself. I know that sounds corny, but we have to start somewhere. Facebook is so huge now! Everyone is asking you to "like" their page, or be their "friend." What about you?

What did you do today that showed yourself some TLC? Maybe some of you went to yoga class. Maybe you took yourself out for lunch. How about taking yourself shopping for that something you have been thinking about for over a week. You understand where I am going here. Our health starts on the inside—how we think, how we feel, what emotions are running through our bodies. It's all connected. If we have "stinkin' thinkin," we are not going to BE WELL. It's that simple!

One of my favorite speakers and teachers, Joyce Meyer, has a whole teaching on "Self Talk." You can find her and download her free podcasts from her website at www.joycemeyer.org. She is hilarious and holds nothing back. If this is tugging at your heart, check it out. If not, share it with someone who needs a little boost.

So in the future, when you hear the negative self-talk start, put an end to it. Think: Would I say those things to my friend? No, so don't say those things to yourself.

Today's Scripture:

"For as he thinks in his heart, so is he."

—Proverbs 23:7 [nkjv]

We have to hold our thoughts captive, especially the negative ones, and give them to God. Otherwise, we start to become the broken record running in our heads.

Let's Pray:

Heavenly Father,

Thank You for loving us so much. Help us to realize truly how much You love us. I pray that You would teach us grace. Teach us how to take care of ourselves no matter what. Teach us that we need to be a priority in our own day. Help us to replace any "stinkin' thinkin" with positive words from You, Lord. I pray for my readers today. May You bless them and meet them where they are. In Jesus' name, Amen!

Lessons Learned Today:

Who are your friends or the support system you call on?

____

____

____

____

What helps comfort you when you are feeling out of balance?

Journal Time:

Write some of the negative thoughts that were running through your head today.

Write some positive thoughts now. My favorite is "I am healthy and I am whole!"

Write about a time when you had just the perfect day. Start from when you woke up until the end of the day. Create the most perfect day.

Now go live it!

DAY 21

Building Blocks

Whoo Hoo! You made it through a full 21-Day cleanse! Some of you are so glad its over; however, some of you may not want this great feeling to stop. Wherever you are, I am so glad you joined me for this cleanse. One thing is for sure, the next time you do a cleanse, it will be much easier. A good cleanse is a great way to reset your body. If you ever get too focused on a food or habit and it starts to take you over, just do a cleanse or a green juice fast. It will help you break the cravings and reset your body's natural metabolism.

I hope you have taken some time to reflect and focus on the one to three things you want to change in your diet. I took a sip of my husband's decaf coffee at the end my of my last cleanse and it tasted completely different than it did on Day One. It tasted horrible, actually! So, many of you may experience similar taste changes. You want to let go of that food or drink as well. I know you all are different today than you were on the first day. I hope you took notes and responded to the journal questions tracking your progress, whether it was good or bad. All progress is growth. Without it, we can't BE what God calls us to be. I hope this journey was a new foundation for you and created BUILDING BLOCKS for your health.

Congratulations to everyone! Whether you were a prayer warrior, or quietly doing your own challenge at home, thank you for lending your hearts and allowing me to share mine. My goal was to show you the health changes that can occur through changing your diet. If you continue on this path of great food for fuel, your body can be unstoppable!

I love and appreciate you all.

If you ever need anything, please do not hesitate to contact me. Keep on going. Remember, YOU WERE MADE TO HEAL!

Today's Scripture:

> "Look to the Lord and ask for His strength. Look to Him all the time."
>
> —1 Chronicles 16:11

Let's Pray:

Heavenly Father,

Thank You for my friend who has just made it through 21 days of disciplined and mindful eating. I pray that You have shown them some areas they can change by letting go of habits that do not serve them nor their body. Lord, thank You for all the blessings and awakening moments they have had. I pray this cleanse catapults them into a new person, from the inside out. In Jesus' precious name, Amen!

Lessons Learned Today:

What did I learn during this process?

____

____

____

____

____

What will I carry with me after today?

How has this experience changed me?

How has this experience brought me closer to God?

Journal Time:

After thinking about the one to three things you want to change in your diet, think about what you want to change in your life.

The New Normal

Now what? What do you do? Do you go back and start eating everything in sight? NO . . . well, maybe one day. (Just kidding) Stay the course! Continue with your protein shakes and fruit. Keep eating vegetables and greens in every meal. Keep leaning toward the 80% plant-based diet, which will keep your body more alkaline. The benefits will prevent many diseases and future illnesses in your body. Slowly reintroduce dairy, caffeine, meat and sugar, but never more than 20% of what you consume. These are big hitters in suppressing your body's natural immune system. The more you limit them, the healthier your body will be.

If you will add at least three things from the program to your new norm, it will make all your hard work worth it! Most of my patients shared that they have felt so amazing, they did not want to stop eating so well. Once you go back to eating carbs, refined sugars, or drinking coffee, you will notice the difference. Since you have successfully cleared those foods from your body, it would be great to see how long you can last in keeping them out of your body.

So my question for you, as we close our cleanse and detox, is: what are three things you can do without for the next three months? Write it down!! Once you write it down, your brain will keep you there on many levels.[10]

Your final piece of homework is to do this detox program every three months, six months or every year. Whatever you think you need. If you start to feel the toxic symptoms coming around again, it's time to reboot your system. You can also do a one-day cleanse by juicing greens with one apple. Drink freshly pressed green juice for three consecutive meals and you will feel amazing. I do that once every couple of weeks. I also do a three-day juice fast when I feel like I have been out of balance with my food and life. These are all great recommendations I share with all my patients. I hope you can adopt some of them.

Here's my hope for you: that you have found a new healthier place to live—a NEW NORMAL. I hope you have surrendered some unhealthy habits so your body will function better and actually HEAL BETTER! I pray that you make your health a priority before you are FORCED to because of a new diagnosis (a.k.a Health Opportunity)!

You were fearfully and wonderfully made by your Creator—God Almighty! I hope this journey has been successful and life changing in many ways. From my heart to yours God Bless!

Appendix A

Grocery List

Fruits:

All fruits are acceptable. If dealing with a health challenge, stick to berries. Berries have the lowest affect on blood sugar.

Don't forget: LENTILS, BROWN or WILD RICE

Bananas	Tangerines
Blueberries	Mango
Strawberries	Peaches
Raspberries	Pear
Pineapples	Plums
Kiwis	Grapes
Oranges	Watermelon (Highest sugar)

Greens: Leafy Veggies

Kale	Red Leaf/Butter lettuce
Collard Greens	Romaine lettuce
Mustard Greens	Endive

Spinach	Escarole
Arugula	Beets

Vegetables:

Anything organic and as much as you can eat! Consume twice as many vegetables as fruit.

Broccoli	Cabbage	Bean Sprouts
Beets	Egg Plant	Leeks
Cauliflower	Garlic	Celery
Mushrooms	Squash	Cucumber
Carrots	Sweet Potatoes (1/2)	Okra
Peppers	Zucchini	Bok Choy

The Extras: Don't Forget

Teas: Dessert teas from Republic of Tea, Numi

Teeccino: Herbal Coffee

Coconut Milk instead of creamer (No sugar if possible)

Mayan Superfoods: Raw Cacao Powder

Raw Cacao Nibs

Almond Butter

Almond Milk or Rice Milk (Unsweetened)

Extra Virgin Oil

Grapeseed Oil

Salsa

Kale Chips

Raw Veggie Dehydrated Crackers—only for Day 11-21 (for emergencies)

LOTS of WATER ready to go![11]

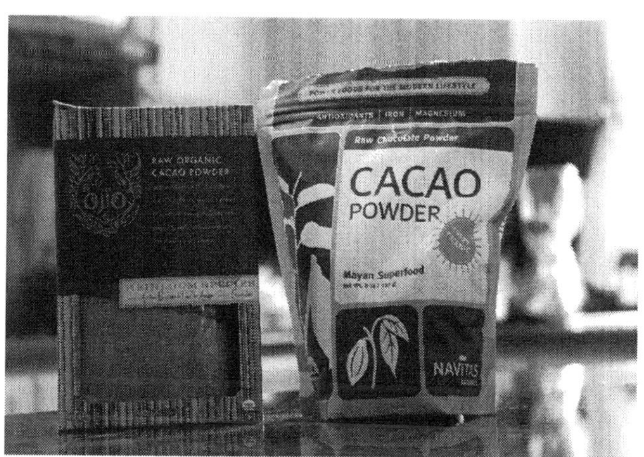

APPENDIX B

The Battle Plan

Daily Routine:

Upon waking, drink water with lemon
(Wheat grass in place of supplement, no food for 1 hour)

Supplements:

*Take SP Cleanse, 7 capsules

20-30 minute transit time

Morning Protein Shake

2-3 scoops of Protein Powder
½ banana
Handful of blueberries/strawberries
1 cup Almond Milk (Unsweetened)
Add a little ice or water to achieve desired thickness
Add 1 tsp. Raw Cacao Powder (if you like chocolate)

Supplements:

*Take SP Gastro-Fiber, 3 capsules

Morning Snack

Veggies or fruit
Green juice
8-10 oz. water . . . lots of water

Supplements:

*Take SP Cleanse, 7 capsules

Lunch

Vegetable soup, lentils, salad
Steamed veggies with brown rice
No meat protein yet! Lots of greens
No dairy dressings, only olive oil and lemon

Supplements:

*Take SP Gastro-Fiber, 3 capsules after lunch

Snack: 3-5pm

Protein shake (Blended at home)
At work-add water to Jay Robb Egg White
Protein powder (chocolate) in a shaker with
1 tsp. of Raw Cacao powder! Delicious!
(Wheat grass-empty stomach no food for 1 hour)
**Only take Egg White Protein or Whey if you have no allergies to milk or egg

Supplements:

*Take SP Cleanse 7 capsules

Dinner:

Veggies and lentils, ½ sweet potato
Lots of water, herbal tea

Supplements:

*Take SP Gastro-Fiber 3 capsules

Dessert Teas

Herbal and caffeine free varieties by Republic of Tea
(My personal favorite is Red Velvet Chocolate)

Dessert/Snack

Fruit, or a spoonful of almond butter with some cacao nibs
Lots of water. Try to sleep on an empty stomach

*Please note: You can use the Whole Food Fiber powder in place of the Gastro-Fiber in order to take less capsules or if you have GI issues already. It easily blends with your smoothie. Your healthcare professional can help you make the right decision for you.

Reminders:

DAY 8, Stop the Cleanse, Add the Green Food, DAY 11, Add Clean Protein (Fish or Meat)

APPENDIX C

Recipes

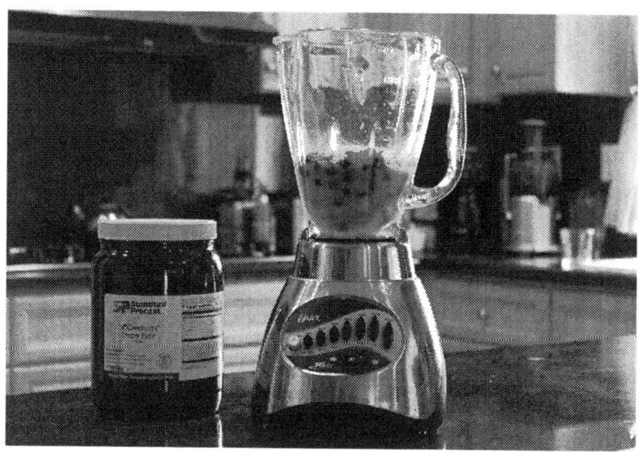

Smoothie Formula:

1-2 scoops of your Protein Powder + ½ banana + berries or other fruit + 1 cup of water or almond milk + handful of greens (spinach or frozen broccoli) = SUCCESS

Add Raw Cacao Powder and Nibs for extra taste and antioxidants.

Smoothies on the Run:

Take a small shaker bottle, add 1 big scoop of Jay Robb

Chocolate protein (Egg White or Whey), 1 teaspoon of

Raw Cacao Powder—Done!

Add ice-cold water when you are ready to drink

Perfect between meetings, or when stuck in the car

I found that Jay Robb is better for the shaker. It blends easier and tastes great on its own without ARTIFICIAL SWEETENERS!!

*Only take Egg White Protein or Whey if you have no allergies to milk or egg

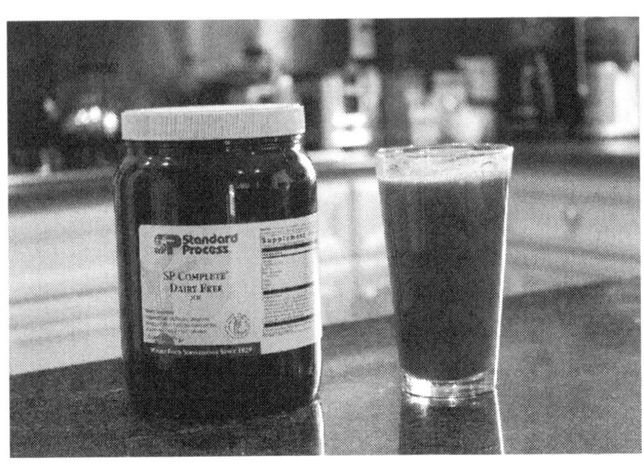

Chocolate Peanut Butter Surprise: a.k.a (3 O'clock fix)

2 scoops of SP Complete-Dairy Free

½ banana

2 Tbsp. of Almond Butter

1 Tbsp. of Cacao Powder

½ cup of water, ice

½ cup of Rice/Almond Milk

Tropical Breeze

2 scoops of protein powder

½ banana

Frozen mangos, pineapples

Juice of an orange

1 cup of water, little ice

Cinnamon Coconut Butter Truffles

¼ cup coconut butter, melted

1 tsp. pure vanilla extract

A pinch or two of salt

1 tsp. ground cinnamon

Combine coconut butter, vanilla extract, and salt. Stir with a spoon until all are combined.

Sprinkle the ground cinnamon on top of the coconut butter mixture and stir until it is fully combined into the mixture.

Place mixture into the fridge for 10-15 minutes to harden enough to roll into balls.

Form coconut butter mixture into 4 equal balls and place on a small dish. Freeze for 10 minutes and enjoy!

Cinnamon Coconut Butter Truffles

¾ cup Almond Butter

1 tsp Pure Vanilla Extract

1/3 cup Shredded Coconut, unsweetened

½ Tbsp Cocoa Powder, Organic

Combine all ingredients in a small mixing bowl. Stir mixture until all ingredients are equally blended together. Form mixture into small balls and place on a parchment lined cookie sheet.

Place in the freezer for 10-15 minutes. Enjoy!

About the Author

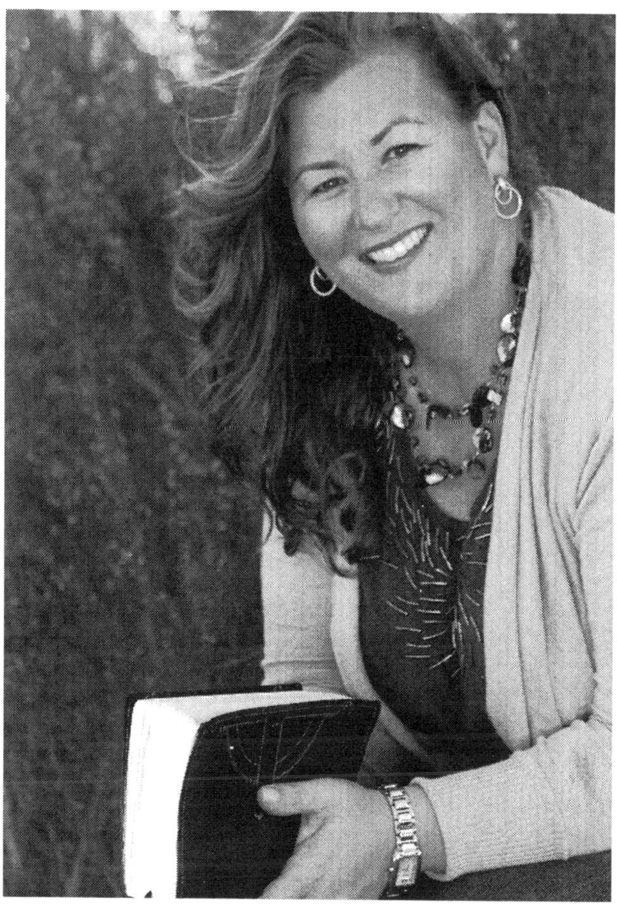

Dr. Angie Welikala graduated from Cleveland Chiropractic College, Los Angeles, December of 1999. She has a Fellowship degree with the International Chiropractic Pediatric Association and specializes in children and pregnant women. She also works with special needs children with Autism and Cerebral Palsy. Dr. Angie was in private practice five years in Moorpark, then took time off to take care of her family and help in her husband's dental practice. She opened up her own Wellness Center in Moorpark CA, in May of 2012. The center provides chiropractic care, massage, nutrition counseling, and yoga classes.

Dr. Angie is also a motivational speaker and loves to inspire and share important health topics with any company or organization. She is very involved with the Proverbs 31 organization and has grown tremendously attending the "She Speaks" events in North Carolina every July.

Dr. Angie is dedicated to her family and she strives to stay focused on what God has called her to do in life. She feels her purpose is to, "love and encourage as many people possible and to live the HEALTH-FILLED life God intended."

Dr. Angie is excited and passionate to share the Word of God with as many people as possible. She loves to share her own imperfections and struggles with other women and men so that all can ultimately grow closer to God and be more like Christ. At the heart of her ministry is Romans 12:8:

> "If your gift is to encourage others, do it! If you have money, share it generously. If God has given you leadership ability, take the responsibility seriously. And if you have a gift for showing kindness to others, do it gladly."

That is her vision and this is where God is leading her.

For more information or to schedule her to speak to your group or organization you can go to www.MadetoHeal.com.

Notes

[1] O'Shea, D.C., Tim. "Journey to the Center of Your Colon." The Doctor Within. 1987. Accessed November 3, 2012.

[2] Anderson, D.C., Greg, "Wellness University", 2011

[3] Environmental Working Group. Accessed November 19, 2012. www.EWG.org.

[4] O'Shea, ibid

[5] The American Heritage Dictionary of the English Language. 4th ed. N.p.: Houghton Mifflin Company, 2009.

[6] Young, Sara. Jesus Calling: 365 Devotions For Kids. Nashville: Thomas Nelson, 2010.

[7] Arterburn, Stephen, and Linda S. Mintle. Lose It for Life. N.p.: Integrity Publishers, 2004

[8] http://www.goodreads.com/quotes/33080-god-loves-you-just-the-way-you-are-but-he

[9] http://www.brainyquote.com/quotes/quotes/r/ralphwaldo107066.html

[10] Klauser, Henriette A. Write It Down, Make It Happen. N.p.: Scribner, 2001.

[11] https://www.standardprocess.com/Products/Standard-Process/Purification-Product-Kit-Gastro-Fiber

25471317R10080

Made in the USA
Charleston, SC
02 January 2014